Mind Your Health, or Mind Your Death

Choose Your Path

A Journey from Autoimmune Disease to
Vibrant Health Without Drugs

Moirar M. Leveille

Table of Contents

Dedication

To my friends and family.

To my ongoing cheerleaders.

To many of you struggling with the symptoms of diseases and diagnosis. May you find inner strength, hope, to be empowered to start your healing journey and gain the confidence to succeed and heal.

MIND YOUR HEALTH

"The type of connection you express to your body determines your health status.

This book is for YOU! It is to help you move on from helplessness to empowerment. It is intended to help you take charge of your health.

No one knows you better than you do. As you become more aware of the beauty of handling your health matters, you will have no fears in asking your health care provider the "what, why, when, where, how" questions that sometimes leave us out of controlling our own health care.

Like many of you, I used to think that my doctors had the answers to my health care needs, so there was no reason to question them. Once I questioned my health care provider and didn't receive an answer to my "what, why, when, where, how" questions, I decided it was time that I do something about it.

When I was first diagnosed with an autoimmune disease over a decade ago, (Hyperthyroid then Graves' disease, and other issues) I can still remember the anguish and the stress dealing with all of the symptoms. I never thought my eyesight would be normal again, I did not know what a regular heartbeat was, I could hear the sound of my heartbeat, and I tried to normalize it. I was not aware that I could have my life back, because I did not know there was a way out.

My deep sense of helplessness made it even worse. Conventional medicine provided no answers to me at that time. From hopelessness was born, a different way of thinking to get empowered or to die. Since I did not want to die yet, I had to be empowered and do everything within my power to get to the root cause of my issues.

I consider myself a lucky one to have believed that all diseases came from imbalances in the body, and by using the functional medicine approach to identify the main source of my imbalances, I became hopeful. My symptoms started to dissipate. I needed to heal from inside out first. Functional medicine opened my view to a comprehensive framework, modern, to understand the complexity of the interconnectedness of the biological system. It provided me a more comprehensive view of the whole system and not just the symptoms.

When I was diagnosed, it absolutely consumed me. I was more worried about the diagnosis than the symptoms. When I was told there was no cure, I was devastated. I became lost, felt helpless, and was desperate. I asked myself, "How come?" How did that happen to me? The doctor must have made a mistake, I asked for a second, third opinion. I wanted to believe I was in a dream, but then reality would creep in.

Every six weeks, I traveled from home to my "God" sorry I meant to say specialist to get the same question and answer from him.

"Mrs. Leveille, how are you today? Everything is looking good, continue with your medication."

Everything looks good, but continue the medication? I was so confused by his answer time after time after time. I was so frustrated. Was I going to feel better, or was I supposed to just accept the life sentence?

At the next appointment, I asked the doctor, "Why am I so sick?" and I told him my side effects.

He rudely turned around and said, "You don't want to take medication forever. You don't want surgery," (because I had the huge bulgy eyes which is a symptom of Graves' disease) "Then what do you want from me, Mrs. Leveille?"

I looked at him and with my tears, and I said to him, "I just want to know why. Why I'm so sick? I'm trying to eat healthily; I don't know what to do, but you're not giving me answers." And I got up that day and I said, "I think we are done now." I took my belongings and put them in my bag. I stood up. With all my anxiety, with all my fears that still come up for me just like they did the first time, I said to myself, "I'm getting out of his office" and I told him, "You'll never see me here again."

That day was his gift to me. "The give of taking full responsibility to manage my health." His words woke me up from my nightmares. Of course, I did not want it. It was too much to handle, it is easier to being told what to do and putting the responsibilities on others. We are not always aware of our power. Sometimes, we live like we are in a coma while life passes us by. I knew I had to take control. So I did. I was scared, but because I took the challenge, now I can be grateful to him for my vitality and my new way of thinking about health.

Making that decision gave me my life back. My health took a complete 360° turn. It was because I incorporated all of the necessary steps, mindfulness, decreasing stress, exercising, using the right approach, including vitamins and nutrients to get all of my energy back. If you ever felt you have lost all power and control over your health matter, your diseases, your fears, others are in control of your destiny, read on and claim your power back. Do not give it away anymore.

You are in control of your vibrancy—of your life, your health, everything. Knowing, if you're not minding your health, you're minding your death. It is just a matter of time you will be bedridden, eating all the food you never dreamed of eating, others will be making all the health decisions on your behalf, and you will have nothing to say about YOU. Isn't that scary? Ok don't stop now, keep on reading to claim your victory over sickness.

OR MIND YOUR DEATH

"Unconscious living is minding death purely."

Early death for individuals is most generally because of sicknesses brought about by smoking, hypertension, high cholesterol, drug abuse, obesity, and physical idleness. Changing your way of life can prevent numerous sicknesses.

A risk factor is something that makes it more probable that you will develop a specific sickness or ailment. Some risk factors, for example, age, sexual orientation, and family, are outside your ability to control. Be that as it may, numerous things that are life-related risk components are especially within your control.

You can drastically lessen your danger of sickness and early death by making a couple of correct way of life changes. Some risk factors that people can control, and change could be obesity, blood pressure, lifestyle, and cholesterol level.

This book, however, will guide you through ways you can mind your health and combat early death. Happy reading.

CHAPTER 1: LIVING DEAD OR BE ALIVE

"Your health status determines if you are Living dead or alive."

How to Live a Healthier Life

People endeavor to be healthier, yet for many individuals, it's truly a struggle. What we've learned is that everyone's perspective on what "being healthy" means is different.

What Being Healthy Really Implies

Our perspective on being healthy is very shallow. For reasons unknown, being healthy is a lifestyle—a method for living. There is no pill that you can take to accomplish an ideal outcome and keep it up until the end of time. It's a lifetime of choices made every single day.

Indeed, you may probably get the body you've always longed for following a couple of difficult long periods of diet and exercise, but if you're not someone bound for the Olympics, we'd wager you'd get tired after a while.

Here is the cool part:

You don't need to do anything radical to live healthier!

You don't need to plunge into anything exhausting, seeking after a change that will stick. You don't need to go full keto (except if that is your 'thing'). You should simply play the Healthy Living Game.

Healthy Living Game:

Level 0

This game, much like life, has levels to it. Everybody begins at Level 0, yet individuals differ en route. Some go on to Levels 5, 10, 20, or 50. Some stay at Level 0.

Everyone advances at their very own rate. Each dimension may contrast from individual to individual.

Let's take a look at a case of what your movement through the positions may be.

Suppose you're starting your voyage to a more beneficial life. And let's say you're currently at Level 0. None of your suppers are home-cooked. Most originate from the window of a drive-through eatery. Rather than carelessly pushing McDonald's cheeseburgers down your throat like a pelican, try this:

Ask yourself...

"What would I be able to do to settle on this choice and make it somewhat more beneficial?"

You don't need to quit going to McDonald's—at least not at Level 0.

In any case, what would you be able to do?

You could...

1. Eat your cheeseburger with one less bun

2.   Request a small rather than a medium (which resembles an enormous at any rate)

3.   Request water rather than a Coke.

By doing only one of these things, you settled on a cognizant choice to carry on with a healthier life. Keep in mind that you—or whoever's with you—might not imagine that is a major ordeal, but it is. Beyond any doubt, despite everything, you're eating inexpensive food, but this time, you've made one little positive development.

Pose to yourself this inquiry with each dinner. A little while later, as it forms a habit, you're out of Level 0 and onto the next.

Level 1

Now you've gotten the hang of eating healthier at your preferred cheap food joints. Since you've aced the cheap food game, you're motivated to make a marginally greater change.

It's noon, and you again ask yourself:

"What would I be able to do to make this choice somewhat more advantageous?"

Rather than McDonald's, you choose to go to Subway. Rather than stacking up on trans-fats and solidified burgers, you get a delightful sandwich and a sack of chips. While absolutely not the exemplification of a "healthy" supper, this is a dramatic contrasted with a week ago!

Also, your supper has 300 fewer calories than your go-to inexpensive burger joint!

Levels 2 & Up

So now, you're feeling super about yourself and have been proceeding to make your outings much more advantageous.

Now you get some meat, some mayonnaise, some sliced cheddar, and some bread to make sandwiches. At that point, you snatch a sack of chips to eat as an afterthought.

Level 2 completed.

So far, your game is going incredible. Particularly on the off chance that you can continue gaining ground unrestricted. But let's face it, life doesn't work that way.

No perspiration. The healthy living game is really made for this sort of living.

It doesn't make a difference what you're doing, what level you're on, or where you're at, the manner in which you carry on with a more beneficial life is by taking a look at your present circumstance and indeed asking yourself...

"What would I be able to do to make this choice somewhat more beneficially?"

For instance, you may be a screwing demigod who eats impeccably "solid" foods in general, however, you additionally need to go out of town for events once per month. This puts a wrench into your arrangements since you can't cook from home while away, particularly not during weekdays.

Have you at any point attempted to eat well while traveling for business? It's damn close to unthinkable.

But maybe you beat this challenge and still carry on. You are beginning to succeed at good choices somewhat with your changed outlook.

Rather than feeling like poo for agreeing to the McDonald's cheeseburger directly outside your plane's door (sorry Ronald, don't intend to continue making you sound like the troublemaker), you can play the more advantageous living game with the cards you were given.

Choose the cheeseburger, but remove the buns.
Avoid the fries.
You know the drill.

It's OK to return a couple of levels on the grounds that truly, you probably won't have a choice. Try not to detest yourself for enjoying a fast, delicious meal since it doesn't work with your new way of life. As you are willing to change your standards you will find, everything works with your new way of living.

This is how you begin to live a life that is beneficial forever.

By taking this to heart, you're not always searching for approaches to eat as solid as would be prudent, you've additionally built up a sound association with your diet—you're OK not being flawless constantly. What's more, that is how life ought to be.

This works with all the things in your life, not simply food.

In opposition to what you may figure, this book isn't just about your diet. Living a more beneficial life is considerably more than that.

The amazing thing about this game is that it can be played anyplace, with pretty much anything.

What's more, when life rattles you, that's ok. Play the more beneficial living game with the cards you have.

Regardless of where you are at this moment, what level you're on, or what you do, in every case you're allowed to play. What's more, it makes you a healthier individual. Go and play and have fun.

CHAPTER 2: HOW TO MIND YOUR HEALTH

"Keep your vitality. A life without health is like a river that is without water."

"Health is wealth. Without health, wealth is wasted". You can't enjoy the pleasure of a happy life without being healthy. You can't achieve your goals if you are sick all the time. The busy lifestyles, schedules, and routines we have today prevent us from keeping a focused eye on our current health. We lose sight of what truly matters. We don't give enough importance to this old meaningful proverb.

According to the World Health Organization, "Health is a state of complete physical, mental and social wellbeing and not merely the absence of disease or infirmity." So, it is better to mind your whole health. You should access the three basic components of entire body wellness. These are your body, your mind, and your soul.

We have to consider them and stay aware of the messages our body is giving to us. Consider them a gift, or a scream for help to support us optimally. We need a beneficial wellness approach to our whole body wellness for a better physical and mental life. If we don't take care of our health, day by day, we get closer to hugging a deadly medical condition. "Oops, too late," I did not see that coming. Well, you have been ignoring all the information your body had given to you such as headaches, low energy, fatigue, low libido, erectile dysfunction, lack of concentration, dizziness, blurred vision, rapid heart rate, hot flashes, and more. These symptoms are reminders that something needs to be taking care of by you, take them seriously, and follow up. Daily, we focus on and give proper care to other things, but don't care for our wellbeing and don't keep a strong and vigorous lifestyle on the priority list because "a healthy lifestyle not only changes your body, it changes your mind, your attitude, and your mood" stated by Gurudev Sri Sri Shankar.

Do you ever think about a better lifestyle? Do you know how to live a quality, healthy life? Have you ever tried for better, medically speaking? Do you ever think of what is essential for your exceptional lifestyle? Most of you will answer NO to these questions. Then you wonder, where is the doctor comes from this diagnosis?

A holistic wellness approach will keep you on a healthy track and will provide a better ability to answer yes to the above questions. Minding your health is not a difficult task, but you have to show passion to your flourishing existence rather than moving and sacrificing yourself naturally. Mind your health for a better life to perform daily tasks well, and enjoy the pleasure of happiness, get fruitful outcomes from what you struggled for, and lot more associated with perfect wellbeing. Holistic health emphasizes the interdependence of the whole body and utilizes these relations for a healthy lifestyle. It empowers you to better treat your medical conditions.

"Our bodies and each system should be treated as a whole, not a collection of its parts. Holistic health addresses the mind, body, and spirit" by Michele Adams. Minding your health is a better approach to wellbeing. In order to do so, you should have enough time to look at the affecting factors, point out the flaws in it, analyze it, and make a plan to get over it. Then, follow up the strategies with passion and consistency.

And don't underestimate the importance of excellent and superior wellness. The above key factors regarding your health not only create a new medical illness in your life but will also impair your ability to cope and positively treat your chronic illnesses.

"Mental health is often missing from public health debates even though it is critical to wellbeing," stated by Diane Abbott. Mental health also has key importance in your whole and hearty wellbeing. Without prime mental health, you can't imagine a splendid lifestyle or physical wellbeing.

So, look around and find what impacts your mind and emotions. Find out how they affect your life. Either they impact it positively or affect it negatively. The more it affects negatively, the more your healthy lifestyle is in danger, and ultimately, the more it is a threat to your goals to success. The Psychological factors related to mental and physical health greatly affect your health. It is better to analyze and find out things as soon as possible that push you into psychological issues such as anxiety, stress, depression, and other psychological illnesses. The good and positive relationship also contribute to your overall state of health.

"Just as a candle cannot burn without fire, men cannot live without a spiritual life," stated by Buddha. The last but not the least thing one should consider for an excellent, beautiful, and elegant healthy life is your spiritual nourishment. Without nourishing your soul, you can't live and enjoy your life. It is best to mind those things that are nourishing your spirit. Determine whether things are driving you to a positive, healthy state or worsening your life, and day to day activities. The soul is directly connected to your mental status and whole wellbeing. If your soul is not well feed, you will get sick, weak, and ill. "The soul always knows what to do to heal itself, the challenge is to silence the mind," stated by Caroline Myss. It is better to nourish it with positive for a superior and aesthetic wellbeing.

George Bernard Shaw stated that "Life is not about finding yourself, life is about creating yourself." Your health not only relies on this, but whatever interferes with these important components will directly impact your comfortable, prosperous, and healthy life. The key to perfect and healthy wellbeing, and the therapy for any medical condition, is solely dependent on these three components. We would be wise to mind our healthy wellbeing to live a splendid and magnificent life.

Here's the rundown:

1. Eat good and balanced foods
2. Base your diet on a lot of foods rich in healthy fats and good carbs
3. Appreciate a lot of fruits and vegetables
4. Decrease salt and sugar consumption

5. Drink a lot of water

6. Keep up a sound body weight

Eat good and balanced foods

For good Health, we need an excess of 40 unique nutrients, and no single food can supply them all. It isn't about a solitary supper, it is about balanced nourishment, that after some time that will have an effect!

High Fat Isn't as Bad as it Sounds

A high-fat lunch could be trailed by a low-fat supper. After a large portion of meat at supper one day, maybe fish ought to be the following day's decision? Base your diet on a lot of foods rich in carbs. I know, it sounds counterproductive from what we have all been told, but it's not.

A large portion of the calories in our diet should originate from nourishments rich in sugars, for example, oats, rice, pasta, potatoes, and bread. It is a smart thought to incorporate at the least, one of these at each dinner. Wholegrain foods, such as wholegrain bread, pasta, and oats, will build our fiber consumption.

Appreciate a lot of fruits and vegetables.

Fruits and vegetables are among the most significant foods for giving us enough nutrients, minerals, and fiber. We should attempt to eat at least 5 servings per day. For instance, a glass of crisp, natural juice at breakfast, maybe an apple and a bit of watermelon as lunch, and a decent amount of various vegetables at every supper.

Reduce salt and sugar consumption.

High salt intake can result in hypertension and increase the danger of cardiovascular disease.

Sugar gives sweetness and an appealing taste, yet sugary foods and beverages are best appreciated with some restraint, as an infrequent treat. Utilizing organic products can help to improve our foods and beverages.

Drink A Lot Of Water.

Grown-ups need to drink at any least 1.5 liters of water daily! Or even more, if it's exceptionally hot, or they are exercising.

Water is the most needed nutrient, obviously. We can utilize tap or mineral water, shining or non-shimmering, plain or seasoned. Natural product juices, tea, sodas, milk, and different beverages, would all be able to be alright - every now and then.

Keep A Healthy Body Weight.

The correct weight for everyone relies upon a number of components, like our sex, stature, age, and other qualities. Being overweight builds the dangers of a wide scope of sicknesses, including diabetes, heart diseases, and cancer.

Overabundant muscle compared to fat originates from eating more than we need. The additional calories can emerge out of any caloric supplement - protein, fat, starch, or alcohol, yet fat is the most thought wellspring of vitality. Exercise causes us to spend that vitality and makes us feel better. The message is sensibly straightforward: on the off chance that we are putting on weight, we have to eat less and be exercising.

CHAPTER 3: HOW ARE YOU MINDING YOUR DEATH?

"Be conscious of health, it says alot about death "

What we often fail to recognize is the small daily things we mindlessly are doing that are killing us. We live unaware of how healthy habits can bring a desire to live vibrantly. We are dying in silence by not taking the time to do what truly matters for our wellbeing. We would rather deal with it when we hear it from our medical doctors who see us just for 15 minutes once a year. We give them full control over our health matter. They are "gods" in our lives, It does not matter if they don't see us for one to five years in our lives, we give them full power to decide, what we should take to be healthy. We completely forget they are humans, not superheroes following us everywhere, knowing everything, I say everything about us. We have a tendency to give that full control to an individual that is as stressed, exhausted, and has all his flaws. We think our doctors have the last say in how we live a healthy and happy life. Even when we know, their words are not making sense based on our lifestyle. When we give our power away, thinking others control our health, we are dying. Within our souls we know what to do. What stops us from doing it? Excuses, justification, forgetfulness, too busy taking care of others' business to get attention. The list goes on and on but let's stop here.

Add your excuses and justifications in this blank space and then commit to a few changes today that will empower you. YOU are in charge from now on, and you are on the right track.

People don't like to discuss death. Be that as it may, having intense discussions about end-of-life care well ahead of time can help dying individuals adapt later on, as indicated by Emily Meier, lead creator of the examination and an analyst who worked in palliative consideration at the University of California San Diego's Morres Cancer Center.

Her exploration recommends that individuals who set their desires in motion and converse with their friends and family about how they want to die can find themselves feeling better despite the unavoidable, and even discover significance in the dying process.

Pain-Free Status

Dying can take quite a while—which here and there implies that patients decide on drugs or expelling life—and emotionally supportive systems suffer because of it.

Emotional Well-Being

Writer and Doctor Atul Gwande abridged prosperity as "The reasons one wishes to be alive" in his ongoing book "Being Mortal".

This may include basic delights like heading off to the ensemble, taking enthusiastic climbs or perusing books. He includes: "At whatever point, genuine disorder or damage strikes your body or mind separately ... What are the trade-offs you are happy to make and not willing to make?"

Kriss Kevorkian, a doctor in anxiety, death and dying, urges those she teaches to compose advance mandates in light of the accompanying question: "What do you need your personal satisfaction to be?"

The emergency clinic setting alone can make tension or contrary emotions in a dying individual, so Kevorkian recommends relatives attempt to make a natural vibe through music, most loved aromas, or discussion, among other choices, or think about whether it's smarter to bring the dying individual home.

Opening Up About Death and Dying

Individuals who transparently talk about death when they are healthy, have a more prominent shot of confronting their own demises with composure. With that in mind, Meier is an enthusiast of death bistros, which have popped up around the country. These casual exchange gatherings expect to help individuals get increasingly open to looking at death, normalizing such discourses over tea or cake. It's where individuals can visit about everything from eternity, to incineration, to burial ceremonies.

Doctors and medical caretakers should likewise defy their very own protection from transparently talking about death, as indicated by Dilip Jeste, a coauthor of the examination and geriatric therapist with the University of California San Diego Stein Institute for Research on Aging. "As doctors, we are instructed to consider how to prolong life," he says. That is the reason dying is seen as a disappointment on our part." While doctors overwhelmingly have confidence in the significance of end-of-life discussions, an ongoing US survey found that almost half (46%) of doctors and pros feel uncertain about how to introduce the topic with their own patients. Maybe, in having a superior comprehension of what a decent passing resembles, doctors and laypeople will be better arranged to help individuals through this last, normal change.

CHAPTER 4: LIVE WITH PASSION

" Be passionate about your health, it will always keep you going."

You probably agree that life is unquestionably an adventure loaded with slopes, valleys, rough roads, and once in a while, smooth roads. Here and there it is unsurprising, and in some cases, it isn't. There might be periods where everything is by all accounts going admirably and different occasions when it appears as though you are a magnet for negative diversions.

Nobody is impenetrable to the downpours of life. We as a whole encounter the preliminaries and mishaps at different occasions, anyway what everybody has is the chance to embrace a positive point of view regardless of what they experience. Your approach will determine the quality of what you allow yourself to feel to empower you or to take you to places that are not helpful for your health.

Let's be honest, intense occasions appear. Individuals will disappoint you. You will encounter misfortune, disappointments, and mishaps. You can concentrate on the negative angles, or you can orientate your attention on the positive perspectives.

You have a decision in each minute about how you react to life—the cards you have don't decide your fate, rather the manner by which you make the appearance. Mentality is foremost as it identifies with whether you carry on with a real existence loaded with enthusiasm and reason or one of disappointment and hatred.

You may have met individuals who have experienced innumerable trials and rehashed mishaps yet still rose with an idealistic frame of mind, particularly towards others, by carrying endowments to those out of luck. They learned important life exercises through their experiences by grasping a positive point of view, paying little interest to the conditions. How would you carry on with an actual existence brimming with energy and reason regardless of when life does not eventuate as arranged?

The manner by which you deal with your feelings decides the dimension of enthusiasm you bring to your background. Feelings are basically vitality in movement. In this manner, if your feelings are principally unconstructive, you are bound by those passionate states that keep you stuck. You are helpless before your negative feelings, as opposed to considering them to be a guidepost directing you toward engaging feelings. Alternately, if your feelings are hopeful, you are carrying on with an actual existence loaded with energy, happiness, harmony, and reason.

Grasp Life With All Your Senses

To carry on with an enthusiastic life, figure out how to grasp your faculties. That is, don't keep down your feelings. Grasp them. Experience them. Process them. And then, let them go. This is a sound method to deal with feelings since feelings need to travel through the body. It has been shown that. Harmful feelings can possibly travel through the body and unleash destruction in a short measure of time.

Seek After That Which You Love

While you may not by any means welcome each part of your life, you unquestionably can seek after that which profoundly resounds with your most profound being. Seek after that which you adore is the hidden message reverberated by the Rumi quote: "Everybody has been made for some specific work, and the craving for that work has been placed in each heart." Life ends up requesting; taking care of work, youngsters, and family obligations and overseeing pressure, so it is crucial to set aside a few minutes to take part in exercises you adore. The sentiments that emerge as you take part in these exercises will revive and animate your soul and empower you to carry on with a real existence brimming with energy and essentialness.

What Do You Want To Do?

Stop at the present time and think about what brings you euphoria and energy. Make a promise to seek after those things all the more as often as possible without becoming involved with the everyday customs of overseeing life. Be brave and intense by rediscovering the delight of doing old things once more. Don't just leave yourself to confinements or burdens which limit your capacity to cooperate with life. Keep in mind: enthusiasm streams where consideration goes.

Discharge Expectations

While arranging and objective-setting, absolutely have their prizes, know that notwithstanding careful arranging, life does not work out as expected. Along these lines, permit space for temporary routes and pit stops on your life's voyage.

Commonly, the most remunerating beneficial encounters show up when you wouldn't dare to hope anymore.

As you discharge desires concerning how life ought to unfurl, you will normally feel more opportunity and energy towards life, since you are never again bound by tense feelings towards future desires. Seen from this point of view, desires are planned feelings of disdain. Absolutely while it is superbly ordinary to have objectives and game plans, I welcome you not to be so unbending with them that you hazard your own, psychological and enthusiastic prosperity.

Unwind. Release. Allow.

Similarly, as PC programming should be redesigned from time to time, be happy to update yourself as well, by accounting for the new. It is said that nature loathes a vacuum and will fill anything left in its place with something new. Change is unavoidable; it is an appropriate procedure of life if your craving is to venture into your brilliance. Discharge the worn out, old projects, viewpoints, convictions, and obsolete projects, which never again serve your potential and internal development. Clear a path for the new, the crisp and imperative extensive vitality, and you will, without a doubt, see energy welcomes its way into your existence with equivalent intensity. Give yourself permission to explore without restrictions, and be opened to reassess to move on with the best options. When these progressions are set aside a few minutes, your point of view and life's conditions will unfurl in the timeliest way. You are qualified to carry on with a real existence of enthusiasm and reason. Concentrate on these key focuses for as brief as thirty days and witness your life change inside a month. Rest guaranteed you can reevaluate yourself in the timeliest way to discover that the increase in your pleasure in life is progressively discernable.

CHAPTER 5: STAY PRESENT NO MATTER WHAT

"The present is the ever moving shadow that divides yesterday from tomorrow."

Figuring out how to remain present takes preparation. It takes everyday practice. The following are a few things you can do each day to enable you to be progressively careful. Begin and end your day right. The beginning of your day has a domino impact on the remainder of your day. It sets the tone for your day. Rather than hurrying to work at the beginning of the day, get up early if you need to and play out your morning schedule. It doesn't need to be contemplation. For you, it could be running or yoga. Anything that causes you to suspend your brain from believing is extraordinary. Your day begins the previous night.

We, as a whole, need to amplify the utilization of our day. In any case, sleeping late will influence our mindset the following morning. We have a tendency to think that it's hard to get up right on time. We think we do not have the self-control to jump right into concerns over our morning schedule, rather than remaining present.

Concentrate On Sense Abilities And Use Them As Updates.

As mind strays during the day, utilize your five senses, touch, smell, hearing, sight and taste, to take you back to your center. What can you keep close to your working environment to keep you grounded? It's about deliberately structuring your working environment with the goal that it urges and reminds you to remain present. Here are a few thoughts:

Touch: You can have little bits of fabrics with various surfaces, bean sacks, or a delicate toy close you.

Smell: You can place blooms, plants, or even espresso powder close to your work area.

Something that has a solid, pleasant smell that makes you focus on it.

Hearing: Light instrumental music, the sound of nature, for example, rain or stream, guided contemplation, and so forth. The best is sound or music that doesn't have any words or verses to them, particularly those that summon compelling feelings.

Sight: Just watch out the window and notice what you see without focusing on the discussion around you. Concentrating exclusively on the hues and the sights makes a difference.

Taste: Take a nibble into a bit of lemon or have an acrid sweet.

The significant thing is to appreciate the sense observations as they are and not pass judgment on them. Simply concentrate on the things and not remark on how delightful they are or not, or how sharp they are or not, and so on. Since when you do, you connect with your brain. It begins to pass judgment and break down what you see through your faculties.

Build up a habit for asking yourself, "What am I doing now?"

We need suggestions to enable us to remain careful, so encircle ourselves with things that help keep us grounded. In any case, we can likewise build up a propensity for self-reminding. I think that it's extremely accommodating to ask myself, "What am I doing now?" or "How am I doing now" followed by a few deep breaths. Doing just that can remind you that you are alive. You have a life, and you are alive.

Asking yourself a question is a progressively delicate way to deal with being careful.

Rather than condemning yourself for not embracing current circumstances, asking yourself a question gives you a similar result without being judgmental. It offers you a chance to pick the best way for yourself. You are not driving yourself to remain present. You are giving yourself a decision. There is a decision between doing your undertaking now or just considering the issue in your mind.

Notwithstanding what you pick, you are being careful and remaining present. Regardless of whether you consider over a wide span of time or not, you are doing it from a position of expectation.

Eat Mindfully

If we are very observant, we can be aware of the relationship between the taste and the feedback we get from the body. The body is the final authority in our food choices, nutrition scientists, or medical doctors.

We can support mindfulness by eating a variety of healthy food and being aware of the feedback from the body.

We all have probably heard the expression, "you are what you eat," but what does this mean exactly? Typically, food is like a fuel to the body, and the kinds of foods and drinks we ingest determine the type of nutrients in our body system and affects how our mind and body are able to function.

- Sugary drinks have empty calories, and they damage the tooth enamel and cause you to gain weight.

- Excess Intake of Caffeine should also be avoided, as it can trigger panic attacks in people with anxiety disorders. Limit your caffeine consumption if you have an anxiety disorder. If you feel like taking caffeine, try tea an alternative. Tea has lower amounts of caffeine than coffee, and it has many antioxidants found in plants that can protect body tissues and prevent the damage of the cell.

- Taking at least about 2 liters of water a day (8 glasses) can prevent dehydration. Studies show that even slight dehydration can cause difficulty concentrating, fatigue, and mood changes, physical effects like thirst, headache, dark or decreased urine, dry skin, dizziness, and constipation.

- Avoid skipping breakfast if you are not fasting. Breakfast is needed to fuel your body, the brain inclusive. Skipping meals can leads to fatigue and brain fog. Incorporate a healthy breakfast into your routine. If you are on a tight schedule in the mornings, grains of a granola bar, yoghurt and fruit can get you a good start for the day.

- Avoid High-fat dairy, refined and fried, sugary foods for dinner and lunch. These series of food have little nutritional value. In addition, they contribute to weight gain and diseases like diabetes, cardiovascular diseases, weight gain, and more. Research has shown that a diet consisting of these kinds of food can increase the risk of depression significantly. Eat a diet that relies on vegetables, fruits, nuts, whole grains, fish, and unsaturated fats (like olive oil). People who choose these kinds of diet are 30% less likely to develop depression than people who consume many meat and dairy products.

Shake Up Your Routine On Occasion.

Having schedules can assist us with saving a ton of time. Be that as it may, it can likewise make our mind anxious and exhausted when it becomes acclimated to everyday practice. An eager personality is bound to discover satisfaction in its own psychological figments, both the past and what's to come.

Every now and then, you have to change your schedules. Focus and acknowledge the present minute. Remaining present is about focusing. You give your complete consideration to whatever errand is within reach. At whatever point you end up diverted from your present undertaking, give uncommon consideration to your contemplations, feelings, and habits. Ask yourself:

What are you fleeing from? What's more, and why?

What are you standing up to? What wouldn't you be able to acknowledge? You can get the hang of something significant about yourself, notwithstanding when you neglect to remain present. Being available at the time doesn't mean you are not safe to pondering the past and what's to come.

Perceiving minutes that you have gone off-track is likewise part of embracing current circumstances. You can possibly find yourself getting occupied when you have mindfulness right now. So you are accomplishing something right.

Rather than censuring yourself for your missteps, acknowledge that you are occupied. Acknowledge that you are fleeing. Acknowledge the present minute as what it seems to be. Also, basically, take your psyche back to the present minute tenderly over and over again until it turns into a habit.

CHAPTER 6: HEALTHY CHOICES

"Take care of your body. It's the only place you have to live."

I t's never past the point where it is possible to begin settling on healthy decisions. By making changes now, you have the ability to cut the danger of getting perpetual diseases.

Change can begin little. By defining practical objectives, you can figure out how to settle on more healthy choices for you, your family, and your environment.

Health doctors realize that your capacity to change your own health habits is influenced by where you live and work, your social background, your pay, your training, your culture, and many other different elements. Yet, there are likewise some risk factors you can't control. You can't control your family medical history, your ethnic foundation, your age, and your sexual orientation. Anyway, by picking a sound way of living, you may lessen your danger of coronary illness and stroke, cancer, diabetes, breathing, and lung infections.

It is difficult to roll out huge improvements. It requires investment to shape new habits. By understanding the progressions you have to make, beginning little and defining practical objectives, you can figure out how to settle on more healthy choices and lessen your risk for ceaseless sickness.

Here are the eight most significant solid decisions you can make:

1. Be a non-smoker and maintain a strategic distance from recycled smoke.
2. Be physically active.
3. Eat balanced and nutrient dense foods.
4. Accomplish a good, balanced weight.
5. Control your blood pressure.
6. Reduce alcohol intake.
7. Lower your stress.
8. Visit a doctor for check-ups once in a while.

CHAPTER 7: TAKE CHARGE OF YOUR HEALTH MATTER

"Take charge of your life! The tides do not command the ship. The sailor does".

Taking control of your Health is basic to a real existence lived well. That is increasingly evident when you're living with a ceaseless health condition. The individuals who do only that will, in general, have better health results Restorative Care Research and Review shows. So regardless of what reasons may have acted as a burden previously, little advances today can at present signify huge changes in your health. Here are health tips to enable you to assume responsibility, beginning at this point.

Get Enough Sleep

Sleep ought to be a top need. The normal grown-up requires seven to eight hours of rest every night. Sleep inadequacy builds your danger of coronary illness, diabetes, cancer, and several other illnesses, the National Institutes of Health reports. Without the sleep you need, all endeavors to assume responsibility for your health lose a portion of their adequacy. That is on the grounds that sleep is the thing that encourages you to recuperate from exercise, think unmistakably, and oversee stress. Lack of sleep can undo the majority of your diligent work with diet and exercise in light of the fact that a drained body can overproduce insulin and ghrelin (the "hunger" hormone). Set up and environment that calm your nervous system and attract sleep.

Schedule A Physical Exam.

Customary health tests are significant for averting sickness and distinguishing issues early. Regular health exams is one of the least difficult approaches to remain diligent over your Health.

As per the Centers for Disease Control and Prevention, your age, Health, family ancestry and way of life decisions all add to deciding how normally you ought to have physical tests, so make certain to examine these components with your doctor to decide how regularly you should come in. Be ready to ask and provide information to your physician, get your answers. A good relationship with your physician matters. Remember, he is a human being like you not as your projected "god" or the person who knows it all.

Be Mindful Of Health Signs

Understanding your fundamental signs, including pulse, heart rate, temperature, and what they mean for your Health can help you proactively sway your prosperity. You can take advantage of doctor visits by carrying a list of questions to ask. Your doctor gathers a great deal of data about your Health, however now and again you may need to speak up.

Improve Your Lifestyle

Assume responsibility for your Health by picking a healthy way of life. Eating a healthy diet and getting ordinary exercise can enable you to keep your weight, glucose level, pulse, and cholesterol level in an optimal range. It is critical to converse with your doctor about what diet and movement are best for you.

CHAPTER 8: THE COST OF YOUR LACK OF DISCIPLINE

"The cost of discipline is always less than the cost of lack of discipline, therefore be disciplined."

To accomplish incredible objectives, you need to be disciplined. Nothing critical is accomplished without discipline.

When you analyze the lives of individuals who have accomplished incredible things, you see this consistent idea: they applied a lot of control in their specific field— whether it is sports, business, academics, and so on.

Numerous individuals have incredible objectives. However, they do not have the control to help them through. They pick the easy way, notwithstanding when it's the incorrect way.

Discipline is the cost of enormity. It's the educational cost you pay to be acknowledged in the world-class school of incredible outcomes.

Be Disciplined in Your Thoughts

Your ideal life is significant. Your mind resembles a greenhouse; it will create in your life what you permit to develop in it. On the off chance that you let, thistles of negative musings multiply in your brain, don't hope to get a heap of extraordinary accomplishments.

Be Disciplined in Your Words

Be cautious with your words; they're amazing. They can make and shape—your life. Simply consider a portion of the words that individuals (for example a parent, an instructor, an ex, a mentor, etc.) have said to you as a child that still affect you today, even after every one of those years. That is the intensity of words. Also, this power can be utilized for good or for bad. Utilize your words for good. Address yourself and others in an engaging manner.

Be Disciplined in Your Actions

Discipline isn't simple; it requests that you make the best decision, notwithstanding when you don't feel like it. That is, you practice your drills, notwithstanding when you don't feel like it. You concentrate notwithstanding when there's an enrapturing show on TV. You chip away at your business, notwithstanding when you'd preferably be playing golf. You sit at the piano and play your scales again and again while your companions are out celebrating. And many other chosen decisions like that and so forth. You do this since you know it's the correct activity to get to your goal.

Your outcomes are extraordinarily affected by your capacity to do what you should be, paying little mind to sentiments. "Restrained activity" gathers speed, and discipline is critical to accomplishing extraordinary objectives. The disciplined individual will outflank the talented one every time. On the off chance that you need to accomplish incredible objectives, you should be restrained in your considerations, words, and moves. You should assume responsibility for your head, your heart, and your hands. Think right, talk right, and do right.

CHAPTER 9: ADDICTION TO YOUR DISEASE

"When you can stop, you don't want to. And when you want to stop, you can't. That's addiction."

A ddiction is an unpredictable disease of the brain and body that includes urgent utilization of at least one substances in spite of genuine Health and social outcomes. Addiction disturbs locales of the mind that are in charge of remuneration, inspiration, learning, judgment, and memory. It harms different body systems just as families, connections, schools, working environments, and neighborhoods.

The Disease Model of Addiction

Addiction is characterized as an infection by most restorative affiliations, including the American Medical Association and the American Society of Addiction Medicine.

Like diabetes, cancer, and coronary illness, addiction is brought about by a blend of social, ecological, and organic components. Hereditary dangers represent only a portion of the probability that an individual will suffer from compulsion.

Addiction includes changes in the working of the mind and body. These progressions might be expedited by dangerous substance use or may pre-exist.

The outcomes of untreated addiction frequently incorporate other physical and emotional well-being issues that require restorative consideration. Whenever left untreated after some time, addiction turns out to be progressively extreme, debilitating, and hazardous.

How Substance Use Changes the Brain

Individuals feel joy when fundamental needs, for example, craving, thirst, and sex are fulfilled. Much of the time, these sentiments of delight are brought about by the arrival of specific synthetic compounds in the brain. Most addictive substances cause the brain to discharge large amounts of these equivalent synthetic substances that are related to delight or reward.

After some time, preceded by the arrival of these synthetic compounds, it causes changes in the brain system associated with remuneration, inspiration, and memory. At the point when these progressions happen, an individual may require the substance to feel ordinary. The individual may likewise encounter exceptional wants or desires for the addictive substance and will keep on utilizing it regardless of hurtful or perilous outcomes. The individual will likewise lean toward the medication to other sound joys and may lose enthusiasm for ordinary life exercises. In the most endless type of sickness, addiction can make an individual quit thinking about their very own or other's prosperity or survival.

These adjustments in the brain can stay for quite a while, even after the individual quits utilizing substances. It is accepted that these progressions may leave those with fixation defenseless against physical and ecological signs that they partner with substance use, otherwise called triggers.

Is Addiction a Chronic Disease?

An interminable illness is a dependable condition that can be controlled, however, not relieved.

Around 25 years old, half of the individuals with a substance use issue seem to have a serious, interminable confusion. For them, addiction is a dynamic, backsliding sickness that requires escalated medications and proceeding with aftercare, observing, and family or companion backing to deal with their recuperation.

Fortunately, even the most serious, interminable type of confusion can be sensible and reversible, as a rule with long haul treatment and kept observing and backing for recuperation.

Are People With Addiction Responsible For Their Actions?

Individuals with addiction ought not to be accused of experiencing the outcome. All individuals settle on decisions about whether to utilize substances. Be that as it may, individuals don't pick how their mind and body react to medications and alcohol, which is the reason individuals with addiction can't control their utilization while others can. Individuals with addiction can at present quit utilizing – it's simply a lot harder than it is for somebody who has not turned out to be addicted.

Individuals with addiction are in charge of looking for treatment and looking after recuperation. Regularly they need the assistance and backing of family, companions, and friends to remain in treatment and increase their odds of survival and recuperation.

CHAPTER 10: SAY GOODBYE TO DISEASES

"Recovery isn't going to be easy. That is the truth. But, if you don't give up, you'll succeed".

Doctors say Focus on Smart Choices. Health, it's the best approach to have a mind-blowing life.

Eat Like a Champion

For good Health, maintain a strategic distance from saturated fats, cholesterol, refined carbs, and sugars and trans-fats.

These foods can cause unending irritation--a typical substantial procedure gone astray that can add to coronary illness, diabetes and considerable cancer.

A little-known truth: diet isn't the most significant factor in deciding your cholesterol level. Just 20 percent of your body's cholesterol originates from your diet, while the other 80 percent is made by your liver. That is the reason it is so difficult to bring down cholesterol through diet alone and why you have to get it checked. It ought to be at an optimal level.

Watch Your Blood Pressure

Do you have hypertension? Regardless of whether you don't think in this way, continue reading. One out of three American grown-ups has hypertension, determined to have a reading over 140/90. Be that as it may, doctors state on the off chance that you are reliably more than 120/80, you additionally have hypertension. Help your heart by keeping your weight and salt intake down and your exercise level up.

Seek after an Ideal Body Mass

Set out to be not quite the same as the normal American, are bound to be larger than grown-ups in some other country. Maintain a healthy weight and abstain from foods that would make you gain weight or get body fat.

Blood Sugar Levels

For good preventive Health, cut back on soft drink, treats, and sugary pastries, which can cause glucose to rise. In the event that you have diabetes, this can harm your heart, kidneys, eyes, and nerves after some time. Overseeing glucose is one of seven measurements for heart Health, as per the American Heart Association. These equivalent measurements make it less inclined to be determined to have cancer.

Get Going

Exercise doesn't need to be in a rec center or organized condition. Doctors state recurrence (how frequently), power (how hard) and time (to what extent) are what matter. Find only 30 minutes, which don't need to be sequential minutes. You could go for short and energetic strolls a few times each day. Or then again complete three 10-minute spurts (or two 15-minute spurts) of movement that fulfill your heart. You want to do a sport or exercise that you truly enjoy, such as dancing, yoga, or anything else that you have fun doing. You do not have to overdo it and increase oxidative stress and cause chronic inflammation.

Stop Smoking

On the off chance that you smoke, there is most likely no other single decision you can make to help your Health more than stopping. While ongoing research found that smokers lose at any least 10 years of future contrasted to individuals who never smoked. It has likewise been discovered that individuals who stopped by age 40 diminish their danger of smoking-related death by 90 percent.

Sleep Soundly

Sleep reestablishes us and affects how we feel. Experience difficulty sleeping? Your diet might be a guilty party. Foods relate straightforwardly to serotonin, a key hormone that — alongside Vitamin B6, B12, and folic corrosive — advances sound sleep. For progressively soothing sleep, focus your diet around the "huge three": complex starches, lean proteins, and unsaturated fats. Exercise, like yoga, can likewise help.

Conclusion

Sound health, health body—we frequently hear this, yet don't do a lot to fuse it in our way of life. Our quick lives have not left us with much decision but to perform various tasks. We, as a whole, are attempting to do as such numerous things in a constrained timespan, and our lives have turned out to be feverish. Which prompts inconsistency in following a solid daily schedule with loads of sound habits. Therefore, our physical and emotional wellness suffer, and we don't feel fit enough to pursue our dreams and complete our daily agendas.

When the stomach growl, we eat. When we feel like we are about to burst, then we stop eating. Our bodies have the ability to recognize and adjust to any changes in the environment and within itself, and sometimes it knows what is best for us without us even knowing. Our bodies can translate biochemical and physiological interactions among cells into sensations through molecules of emotion. Consuming appropriate combination of both primary and secondary compounds results in benefits. Eating excess primary or secondary compounds enforces physiological costs, which is experienced as dissatisfaction and a disliking the flavours of the foods. All these responses change as the cells and organ systems in our body gently guide our choices to meet their collective needs.

As per an English adage, "A healthy mind lives in a healthy body." Even if the body isn't sound, the impacts of this condition won't be lasting given the brain isn't permitted to get influenced.

We should not overlook that "Health is Wealth." If we don't deal with our physical Health, our psychological well-being will consequently suffer. Along these lines, eat on schedule; rest on schedule; do some exercise; take some little breaks; seek after your side interest to adjust yourself; and move towards a solid way of life and a more advantageous "YOU."

Minding your health is possible

Minding your health, it's a holistic experience, a guided own spiritual journey. You are not powerless regarding your health matter, by making simple, consistent changes to leave a happy life you become in control of your vibrancy. Leaving a healthy life is a right, not a privilege, magic, or luck reserved for a special group.

You are in charge of living without the many imbalances or diseases on earth. Your body is capable of dealing with your daily challenges if you are connected, aware, and sensitive to your needs.

Many steps might be needed to take into consideration. Be steady, and no matter what do not give up. Move away from diseases and lean towards wellness. If you feel you are healthy or still alive by chance, reassess, and make some necessary changes to take your health concerns in control. Just know, your diagnosis is not a death sentence, this is just a name given to a collection of symptoms.

Most chronic diseases are not only reversible but also preventable by using an individualized approach to managing stress, exercising, good nutrition, and diet. Your lifestyle contributes to your wellness or illness journey. The key is to establish a balance and get educated throughout your health journey. Do not speed the process of your death by living unaware of your power.

" The part can never be well, unless the whole is well." Plato

YOUR HEALTH MATTERS...
DO SOMETHING ABOUT IT.